Type 2 Dia

Natural Treatments That Will Help Prevent and Reverse Diabetes

By: Wendy Owen HH Dip (H.H.T)

ISBN – 978-1494906917

Reviews

Reading this book is a wake-up call for me as I'm now in my 40s, and sedentary lifestyle have slowly begun to crept in. I loved the holistic manner in which Ms. Owen approached the subject of curing Type 2 Diabetes naturally. From the simple, jargon free introduction to what Type 2 diabetes is, to signs & symptoms to be aware of, to ways of preventing, managing and reversing this lifestyle disease.

I especially enjoyed the chapter on exercise and natural remedies. I was pleasantly surprised to find one of my favorite herb - cinnamon - contains natural compounds that help balance blood glucose.

Finally, I really appreciate the "Points to take away" at the end of each chapter - a succinct summary of important points to remember.

Adrian Ling

I just finished reading Type 2 Diabetes Cure. I like the holistic approach of the author and the way in which the topic - Type 2 Diabetes is covered thoroughly in the book.

The book opens up with a clear distinction between Type 1 and Type 2 diabetes. It covers the causes of Type 2 diabetes, the symptoms, current medication (what the various medication do and their side effects),how to manage and reverse Type 2 diabetes naturally, the role of natural supplements and which sweeteners to avoid.

The book is well written in everyday language making it easy to read and understand. I like the pictures in the book - each one drives home a vital point.

Good news - Type 2 Diabetes can be reversed and this book shows you - how!

Sarah Lincoln

Having had three diabetic cats--all of whom were overweight and all of whom were initially put on insulin until we learned about diet management--I am a firm believer in how a change in diet can have a very positive effect on controlling and even reversing Type 2 diabetes. (Two of my three insulin dependent cats were able to go off of all medication with a change in diet as recommended by our veterinarian, and the third while he still needed oral medication no longer had to have insulin shots) This book takes a responsible tone towards explaining the differences between Type 1 and Type 2 diabetes, symptoms of diabetes to watch out for, and how to manage diabetes through diet. The book is careful to state that while symptoms of Type 2 Diabetes (only) can often be reversed through the suggestions she makes, that it is important to maintain your medication regime as prescribed by your doctor and should you be diagnosed with diabetes to work with your doctor to get the best results from this diet program.

The approach Ms. Owen takes towards explaining how diabetes works and how diet affects diabetes is straightforward and very easy to understand. I thought I had known a fair amount about diabetes from having had family members, friends, and cats with the disease, but this book really taught me even more about the disease including about diabetes medications, what symptoms to watch for (I hadn't known about black skin in the creases), and most importantly, how to eat a diet that will help you not only manage your diabetes, but also do so in a way that keeps the joy in food! The book offers helpful tips and great resources to explore so that you can eat safely and happily. And in addition to diet suggestions, you also get lots of great techniques to adjust your emotional relationship with stress and food. In short, this is a very helpful book that I'm going to be lending right away to my mom who is prediabetic and a number of my diabetic friends as a reference! Great book!

Carla Davis

Disclaimer

Please note that the author is not a medical doctor or a practitioner in the conventional medical field. Instead the author has a diploma in Holistic Health Therapy.

The information in this book is provided for informational purposes only and is not a substitute for professional medical advice. The author makes no legal claims, express or implied. Readers are advised to do their own due diligence when it comes to making medical decisions concerning their health. The material here provided is not intended to replace the advice of a qualified physician.

The author assumes no responsibility for the loss or damage caused, or allegedly caused, directly or indirectly by the use of information contained in this book. The author and publisher specifically disclaim any liability incurred from the use or application of the contents of this book.

Table of Contents

Introduction

Are you sick of painful glucose tests? Are you sick of having to buy expensive diabetes drugs? Do you just want to go back to a normal life without diabetes?

Well now you can.

Maybe you're reading this because you've just been diagnosed with type 2 diabetes. Maybe you've noticed some weird symptoms lately and you're afraid you may have diabetes. Or maybe you're just interested in how to prevent it. Whatever the situation, I have written this with you in mind, so that you can discover how to:

- Reverse your type 2 diabetes
- Understand your symptoms and get the shove you need to get tested, or...
- Dramatically improve your health to the point where you will never become a diabetes statistic

Please note than we are not discussing type 1 diabetes here. That is a completely different disease. In type 1 diabetes the pancreas isn't able to produce insulin. Type 1 diabetes is not caused by lifestyle and type 1 diabetics need to take insulin every day.

Did you know that type 2 diabetes used to be called "adult onset" diabetes? This was because it used to affect older, less healthy individuals. Now teenagers and even children are succumbing to this disease. You could say it's fast becoming an epidemic.

What has changed so much in the last few years for this to have happened? Our lifestyles have become far busier, we are cooking fewer meals at home, our children are parked in front of the computer or the television instead of running around in the sunshine and we are suffering with a lot more stress.

Of course there are drugs especially manufactured to "manage" this type of diabetes. Certainly you can stay on these drugs for the rest of your life if you so choose. Will they cure diabetes? Absolutely not! Only you can cure yourself by taking responsibility for your health from now on and making a commitment to a long and healthy life.

Are you with me? Let's go!

How the Heck Did I End Up With Diabetes?

How is diabetes caused?

I remember listening to my mom, many years ago, talking about a friend of hers who had "sugar-diabetes". I asked her what it was and she replied, "It's a disease you can get when you're older." Being a rather inquisitive kid I asked, "How do you get it? Is it from eating sugar?"

"Oh no!" she replied, "It's a lot more complicated than that."

The funny thing is, we were both right. Diabetes is complicated, but yes, eating sugar can cause weight gain which is a major cause of diabetes type 2.

Type 2 diabetes is mainly a lifestyle disease. In fact you could say it's a disease of our affluent society. The disease is far less prevalent in the third world where food can be scarce and people have no access to processed food.

Type 1 diabetes is caused by an organ called the *pancreas* failing to make sufficient insulin. Type 1 patients have to use supplemental insulin – usually in the form of an injection – every day of their lives. Type 1 is generally referred to as an *auto immune* disease where the small islet cells have been damaged by the body's own immune system.

However type 2 is caused by several factors:

Obesity

It is possible for a person of normal weight to develop diabetes. After all, belly fat can form on a slim frame. However it is less common. Generally, those most at risk of diabetes are overweight or obese.

Lack of exercise

Exercise benefits people with diabetes in several ways. It helps the cells use insulin, it helps with weight loss and it's great for all round good health.

The above are the main risk factors. There are indeed other risk factors for type 2 diabetes. If you have been diagnosed as pre-diabetic or are simply trying to avoid developing diabetes, see how many of these describe your situation. You may be able to address some of them to lower your risk.

Ethnicity

Some races tend to develop diabetes more often than others. These include Hispanics, Africans and Asians. This tends to support the genetic cause of diabetics. If you fit into one of these groups it doesn't mean you will develop type 2 diabetes, you can avoid it by practicing healthy eating and lifestyle practices.

Age

As we get older we are at risk for many diseases, unfortunately. Of course type 2 diabetes is no exception. Generally the risk increases in people who are over forty five years old.

Genetics

If your parents, grandparents or siblings have diabetes, then you could be at greater risk. This could also be because people in a family unit tend to eat the same foods in the same quantities. They also have either a love of exercise, or hate it like the plague!

High serum levels of triglycerides

High triglycerides in the bloodstream are both a risk factor for diabetes and a component in metabolic syndrome (pre-diabetes). Triglycerides are a type of fat and we all have them in our blood. However levels over 150 are considered high.

High triglycerides can also be a symptom of kidney disease or an under active thyroid, so should be investigated.

High blood pressure

Blood pressure levels over 140/90 mmHg are considered high. There are many natural ways to lower blood pressure, such as herbal remedies and stress reduction.

Low levels of HDL cholesterol, or *hypoalphalipoproteinemia* – (don't even try to pronounce this!)

Cholesterol consists of two different types, HDL or good cholesterol and LDL or the bad stuff! Type 2 diabetics tend to display lower levels of HDL and higher levels of LDL which may increase risks of heart disease.

High consumption of alcohol

Do you drink more than 2 standard alcoholic drinks a day? Do you drink every day without ever missing a day? This is putting you at risk of diabetes. Alcohol has a direct effect on glucose levels. Sweet wines contain more sugar which can raise levels, while beer has a high carbohydrate count that can also cause levels to rise quickly.

You can get low carbohydrate beer which is better, but it still contains a certain level of carbohydrate. Wine drinkers are better off with a glass of dry wine.

Gestational diabetes

If you have previously had this disease while pregnant, this can mean you are at increased risk. Nothing you can do about this of course, except be aware that the risk is there.

There are steps you can take to lower your risks if you fit into one or more of the above categories, so stay with me.

Points to take away:

1) The primary causes of diabetes are obesity and a sedentary lifestyle (no exercise)

2) Although there are other risk factors, all these can be overcome - type 2 diabetes is not compulsory!

What Symptoms Should I Look For?

Are you at risk?

You may be worried that you have type 2 diabetes. If you're overweight and have some of the risk factors, you may be wondering what symptoms you should be watching for.

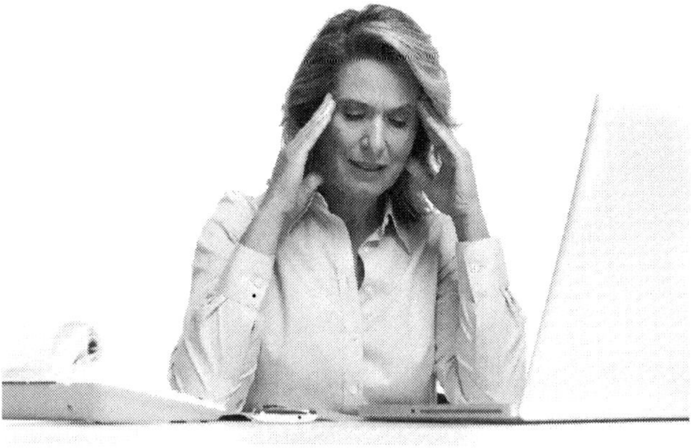

The body of a type 2 diabetic has built up a condition called insulin resistance. In the early stages, the pancreas will actually work overtime to produce more insulin to try and counteract the effects of the insulin resistance, but eventually diabetes will take over and the pancreas just cannot keep up with the demand. Insulin resistance means the cells can't use insulin to absorb glucose to produce energy.

When this occurs, the sugar levels in the blood become over saturated leading to *hyperglycaemia*. Without the insulin breaking down the sugars into energy, this glucose remains in the blood causing all sorts of problems. At first, the body's cells just start to starve for energy. But over time, damage to the body can become quite severe.

Overall, there are many symptoms of type 2 diabetes that can often go unnoticed for years, leading to horrible complications down the line. As such, it is important for each and every person to be aware of the symptoms of type 2 diabetes so they can protect themselves from suffering and seek the proper help that they need should the symptoms develop.

Thirst and Urination: When the overabundant build-up of sugar is coursing through the body, it will actually cause fluid in the surrounding tissues to be pulled into the blood stream like a leech sucking on a leg. When this happens, the body slowly becomes dehydrated, leading to increased thirstiness. As a person constantly drinks more and more to combat this, they will also find themselves taking more trips to the bathroom to urinate.

Hunger: Because the insulin isn't able to do its job in the body, the body's cells are not getting enough energy from the glucose breaking down. This means that your body is literally starving for energy. When the bodies organs aren't getting enough energy, the brain sends a signal to the stomach to trigger intense hunger as a last ditch effort to increase sugar intake.

Weight Loss: This is one of the more obvious symptoms that point towards type 2 diabetes. If you haven't changed your eating or exercise habits and you find yourself losing weight, *then it's a sure sign of diabetes*. The reason for this is that since the sugar cannot be broken down in the body for energy, it is simply expelled in the urine. Instead, the body will target fat cells and muscle cells to use for energy which triggers weight loss, a very unhealthy one at that. This is not a good way to lose weight!

Chronic Fatigue: Naturally, since the body isn't getting the proper energy it needs, anyone suffering from type 2 diabetes becomes very tired all of the time for seemingly no reason. A lot of sufferers will also find themselves easily irritated at the slightest incident.

Visual Impairment: As the blood sugar levels reach even higher and higher saturation points while the insulin struggles to do its job, the sugar will actually leech the fluid from the lenses in the eyes. This will cause blurry vision. The effect is mild at first, and may be corrected with a simple trip to the eye doctor. But as symptoms move forward, it will be painfully obvious that something else is wrong.

The Wound That Just Won't Heal: A very common symptom of type 2 diabetes is having even minor cuts or bacterial infections that just won't heal or go away. This is mostly because white blood cells have a harder time navigating to the source of the injury and take a longer time to do their job because of the high blood glucose. If there is a cut that you've had for ages no matter how well you've been treating it, it may be time to see a doctor.

Dark Skin: Insulin resistance sometimes shows itself in strange ways, one of which is areas of dark skin in the folds or creases in the body. They usually appear around the neck or the armpits, and are a warning of possible diabetes. Itchy skin on those who don't normally experience it can also signal diabetes.

As anyone can see, some of the symptoms of diabetes are hard to pinpoint. This is because there are *other health issues that can cause similar symptoms*. Others, however, are enough to send red flags up for anyone with an eye out for potential health problems. If you have any of these symptoms and have yet to seek treatment, do so today. It could mean a longer, and healthier, life for you.

Points to take away:

1) Symptoms of diabetes can easily be confused with symptoms of other disorders.

2) Losing weight for no apparent reason is a reliable sign of diabetes. However be aware that not all diabetics lose weight.

What Will Happen if I Do Nothing?

"I can't really deal with this right now; I might worry about it when I'm not so busy..."

Trust me, this is not an option. Here's why...

There are hundreds of thousands of people running around today that already have developed pre-diabetes and diabetes. These folk are either completely unaware of the health risk hanging over them, or they are in complete denial and don't want to accept they have a health problem. (I actually have a friend who was in denial for almost a year). So what will happen if diabetes is left untreated? Here's the plain unvarnished truth.

As we already know, the failure of the cells to absorb glucose leads to an enormous amount of glucose circulating around in the blood vessels. The glucose molecules then attach themselves to the body's organs, such as the heart, kidneys, eyes, skin and even the blood vessels themselves. This process is known as *glycation*. This over-abundance of glucose can also affect the immune system.

Kidneys -

In a healthy body, the kidneys filter the blood, ridding it of metabolic wastes such as uric acid. When the kidneys have been damaged by uncontrolled glucose levels, kidney disease (*Nephropathy*) can result. Untreated diabetes is one of the most common causes of kidney failure today. Almost half of all kidney failures are caused by rampant glucose levels.

What happens when the kidneys fail? The only way someone with total kidney failure can be kept alive is through *haemodialysis*. The patient is attached to a dialysis machine via an artery in the arm. The blood is filtered through the machine and returned through a vein. This involves an enormous amount of time spent sitting around in a hospital or clinic several times a week.

A kidney transplant is the only way to avoid dialysis once the kidneys have ceased functioning.

Eyes –

Glucose in the bloodstream can cause a disease called Retinal Disease or *Retinopathy*. The retina is the part of eye that reflects light and sends images to the brain allowing us to "see".

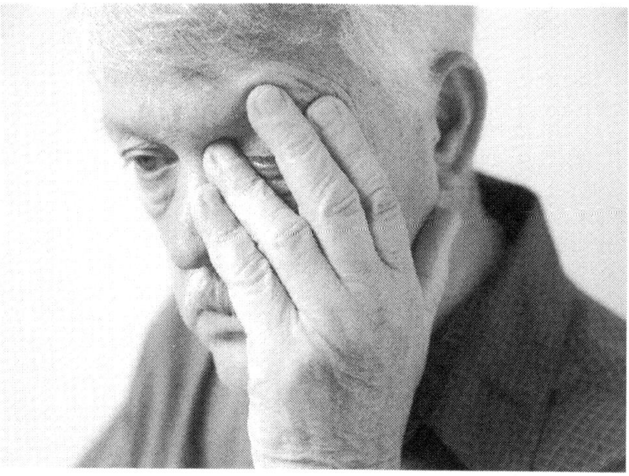

Retinopathy is a leading cause of blindness. Tiny blood vessels in the retina burst and block proper blood flow. This causes inflammation in the retina. The biggest danger of retinopathy is that it can creep up on you without displaying any symptoms. By the time you notice any pain or blurred vision, the damage is already under way.

Laser surgery can repair the damage done by retinal disease to some extent, but is most successful in the early stages of the disease. This is why an eye test for diabetics is so important.

Heart -

Of all the deaths caused by diabetes, up to 75% are caused by heart disease and stroke. People with diabetes are four times more likely to suffer with heart disease. Recent studies have also shown that controlling blood glucose with drugs does NOT reduce this risk. This could be because of other risk factors that come along with diabetes, apart from high glucose levels.

* This is based on studies – ACCORD in the USA, UKPDS in the UK and ADVANCE in Australia. These were performed on many thousands of participants who had type 2 diabetes. The studies found that, despite stringent lowering of blood glucose levels using insulin and other drugs, the incidence

of heart attack did not decrease, but actually rose slightly.

High blood pressure, obesity, high LDL cholesterol levels and high triglyceride levels tend to be more prevalent in diabetics and could be the reason for this increased risk.

There are studies that have been done on this both in the US and Australia *

http://www.diabetes.org/for-media/2010/mixed-results-from-accord-2010.html

Other awful side effects of diabetes...
Nerve pain - (*diabetic neuropathy*)

According to a couple of diabetic people I know, nerve pain is the worst of all the problems they have had to encounter since they became diabetic. There are basically two types of nerve disorders caused by diabetes; sensory loss, in which there is numbness or tingling in the extremities such as the hands and feet, or burning pain in the same areas. Both types of neuropathy are caused by nerve damage and can also cause weakness and muscle wasting.

Neuropathy can affect up to 70% of diabetics and if untreated can lead to amputation.

More frequent infections -
Infections seem to strike the diabetic person more frequently and be harder to get rid of. This is largely due to a depressed immune system. Typical infections include yeast infection or colds and flu.

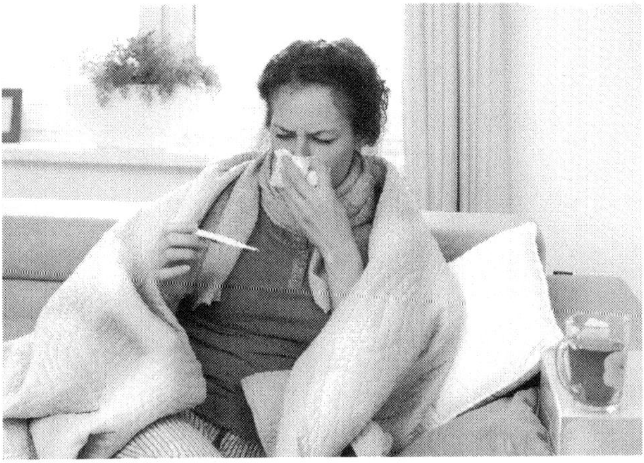

However the skin seems to be the major target for infections that are hard to heal. Abscesses, rashes and fungal infections are especially problematic as they can penetrate the blood stream and become life threatening. The skin is thought to be the organ most at risk for diabetes induced infections, due to damage of the small peripheral blood vessels near the skin's surface.

The above are the main complications of diabetes. As you can see this disease affects the whole body negatively. I hope this chapter gives you the inspiration you need to turn your life around. The good news is you don't have to experience any of the debilitating symptoms listed above.

Type 2 diabetes is curable and we're going to start doing that later in this book.

"Desire is the starting point of all achievement, not a hope, not a wish, but a keen pulsating desire which transcends everything." - Napoleon Hill

Points to take away:

1) If diabetes is left unchecked it will destroy certain organs, nerves and blood vessels.

2) Heart disease, caused by diabetes can't be cured by merely controlling glucose levels. The diabetes itself needs to be reversed for the heart to regain its former health.

The Difference between Pre-Diabetes and Diabetes

What is pre-diabetes?

Pre-diabetes is also known as *metabolic syndrome* and it affects thousands of people today who are blissfully unaware that they have this health issue hanging over them. So what is pre-diabetes?

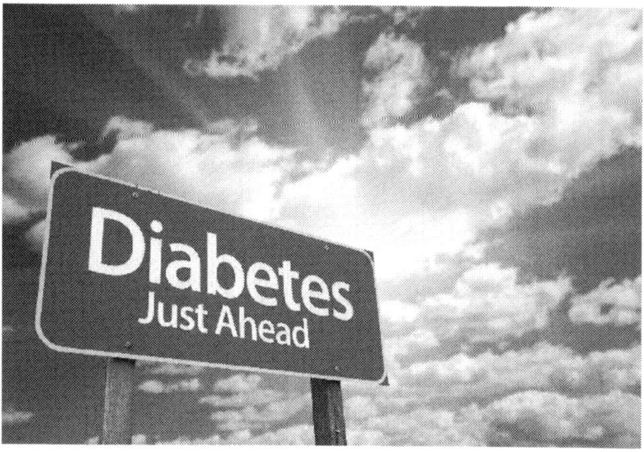

Nobody suddenly becomes diabetic overnight. Excess glucose in the blood stream does its damage very gradually and this is part of the reason why most people are unaware of the condition. It creeps up insidiously, but our body is changing even if we can't see it. Here's what happens...

Almost 25% of the US population over 50 today could be pre-diabetic. That's a startling number of people and it will only rise with time. The difference between pre-diabetes and diabetes itself is simply one of numbers. In other words, if you're pre-diabetic and you continue to do the things you've always done, you will soon be a statistic of diabetes.

Here is a definition of metabolic syndrome:

- Excess belly fat – excess fat around the tummy area is more dangerous than fat around the hips or thighs. This is commonly referred to as the apple body shape.
- High insulin levels.
- High levels of inflammation in the body.
- High blood pressure.
- A preference for highly processed foods.
- High LDL cholesterol levels and low HDL levels.

- High triglycerides.
- People who don't like exercise.

The best and fastest way to reverse yourself out of this condition is to get rid of the belly fat. I'll explain why:

The accumulation of fat (visceral adipose tissue) around the waist and stomach is much more dangerous than fat elsewhere on the body that normally sits just under the skin. Firstly this type of fat doesn't just sit neatly on your belly. It also surrounds vital organs such as the heart and liver. This can interfere with the functioning of these organs.

Belly fat itself actually behaves like an organ in the body. It releases inflammatory substances and hormones putting you at risk for all sorts of diseases, namely high blood pressure, diabetes, stroke and heart disease.

Belly fat contains two types of substances called *adipocytokines*. For simplicity's sake we'll call them good and bad adipocytokines. In a normal weight person with a small amount of visceral fat, these two adipocytokines balance each other out quite nicely. However as belly fat increases in volume, more of the bad guys are secreted and less of the good.

Belly fat tends to break down into fatty acids which the liver attempts to neutralize. This can lead to high triglycerides and LDL cholesterol. This inevitably sets the stage for inflammation and insulin resistance.

So how do we get rid of belly fat? Food! - Yes I'm sure you're groaning at this point! However it's not as simple as eating less. It's about what and how you eat too. We'll get into that in a later chapter.

Points to take away:

1) Pre-diabetes is a warning sign for full blown diabetes.

2) Belly fat is the most dangerous fat in the body.

Why Can't I Just Take the Medication?

Diabetes type 2 medications and their side effects

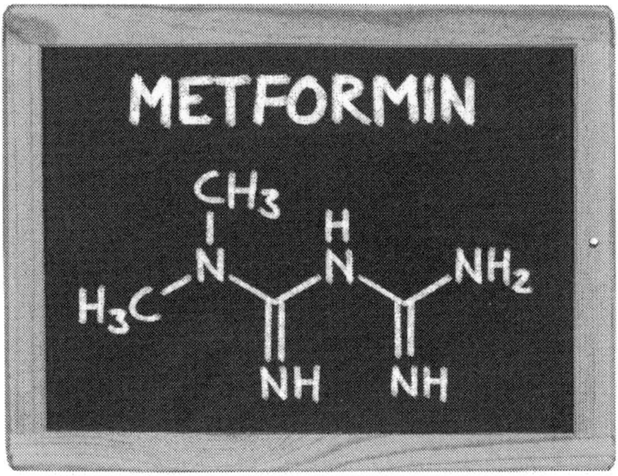

You can just take the medication, but bear in mind, diabetes can be progressive. This means you may need stronger medications next year and the year after. Add to that the cost of these medications and the time consuming blood sugar testing... Nah! Let's get rid of it instead!

However, despite our best efforts, there are a minority of type 2 diabetics that need to take some medication. These folks do not suffer so much with insulin sensitivity as *lack* of insulin.

You need to know what's in that medication you're taking. Here's the drill...

Common Diabetes Medicines and Their Side Effects:

If you have just been diagnosed with diabetes, your doctor may have put you on some type of diabetes medication. There are different types of medications for type 2 diabetes and we'll look at the most common ones here. It's important to know what your medication is actually doing for you and what, if any, side affects you can expect from it.

The type of medication used generally depends on the severity of disease and the person's individual response to the medication.

Unfortunately, most all of these medications have some side effects. A well-known diabetes medication called *Avandia* was withdrawn from sale in 2011, due to increased risks of heart attack in patients. Here are some of the more common side effects from these commonly used drugs.

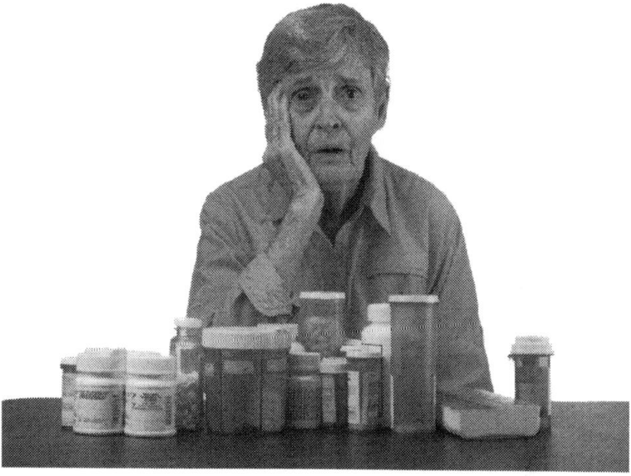

The first class of diabetes medications we will examine are the *Biguanides,* which mainly include *Metformin* and a number of extended release derivations (commonly sold under the brand *Glucophage*). These have a dual action; they reduce the amount of glucose released from stores in the liver and increase the uptake of glucose by the cells, thereby reducing insulin resistance.

Common side effects of these medications include various gastrointestinal problems such as bloating, gas, diarrhea, upset stomach, and poor appetite. These usually hit near the start of the therapy and are best minimized by taking the drug with food. One rare, but important, side effect is *acidosis* which tends to occur in people with poor liver function.

The *sulfonylureas* are also very commonly used to treat diabetes. Common brand names are *Diabinese, Amaryl, Glucotrol,* and *Glipizide.* These medications work to stimulate the production of insulin after a person has finished eating. As one might imagine in a product that stimulates insulin release, low blood sugar is a potential side effect of this drug. Others include skin rash, upset stomach, and irritability.

Thiazolidinediones are also used to treat diabetes with the most well-known example being *Actos.* This class of compounds works by directly improving insulin sensitivity. The major side effect from these medications is fluid retention and swelling. The most serious problem in taking this medicine long term is the increased risk of congestive heart failure.

Meglitinides are another class of medications commonly used. *Prandin* is the classic example, and this drug works by stimulating the release of insulin right after a meal, like the *sulfonylureas*. These differ in that their release is confined to right after the meal is eaten, with no lagging effect for hours afterward. As with the sulfonylureas, the main problem with this drug is the potential to cause lower blood glucose levels. However, due to their shorter action, the danger is not as acute. It's important that this drug be taken with meals (and only with meals) in order for it to work properly.

A nearly identical profile is seen for another class of drugs, the *D-phenylalanine* derivatives. *Starlix* is a commercially available drug in this class.

DPP-4 Inhibitors are a relatively new class of oral medication diagnosed for type 2 diabetes. These have a duel effect of better normalizing the level of insulin after food is eaten and also reducing the body's production of glucose. *Januvia, Onglyza,* and *Tradjenta* are some brands that fall within this particular class of medication. The good news about these medications is that they do not have the risk of causing low blood glucose levels.

However, there are a variety of other side effects. These include gastrointestinal symptoms such as diarrhea and stomach pain. People taking these drugs are also at risk for sore throat, stuffy nose, and upper respiratory infections.

Alpha-glucosidase inhibitors are also used in diabetes treatment. *Precose* and *Glyset* are the two brands associated with this class of medication. These work to slow the absorption of the carbohydrates into your blood stream after you eat, thereby indirectly avoiding an insulin spike. As one might expect, there are gastrointestinal side effects with this drug which include upset stomach, abdominal pain, diarrhea, and gas. However these side effects typically go away after a few weeks of taking the drug.

Bile acid sequestrants are a class of drugs that are less commonly used. *Welchol* (marketed alternatively as *Cholestagel* or *Lodalis*) is the main medication in this class. These are weak inhibitors of LDL cholesterol levels in the blood stream by preventing the release of LDL from the liver. These are often used in combination with medications such as those listed above that regulate glucose metabolism. The side effects are relatively minor and mainly gastrointestinal in nature: constipation, gas, nausea, heartburn, and diarrhea. They can also cause headaches. Doctors must also be careful in prescribing these drugs as there are a number of common drug to drug interactions known.

Due to the fact there are several of the above medications used in combination, the pharmaceutical industry has developed a large number of combination pills to provide more convenient dosing. Examples include Metformin combinations with Glucotrol (*Metaglip*), Januvia (*Janumet*), Onglyza (*kombiglyze*), and Actos (*Actoplus Met*). For each of these drugs the side effect profile is pretty much the same as you would expect from the two drugs taken separately.

As you can see there are many choices and if one drug does not suit an individual, another in the same or different class may be substituted.

However the question you need to ask is this. "Why spend a lot of money on a drug with potential side effects when you can reverse diabetes with diet and lifestyle?"

Points to take away:

1) Drugs have side effects; however don't stop taking prescribed drugs without the advice of your doctor.

2) If you have to take a drug for type 2 diabetes, learn all that you can about it. If the drug is having side effects, you may be able to change to another which suits you better.

Ok - So Where Do I Start?

Standard Tests for Diagnosing Type 2 Diabetes

As type 2 diabetes can develop at any age, it's important to know just what tests are going to be performed to determine what type of diabetes you may have. Overall, once diabetes is suspected, there are four basic tests that your doctor will administer to determine if you actually have diabetes. No they're not fun but *soooo* important!

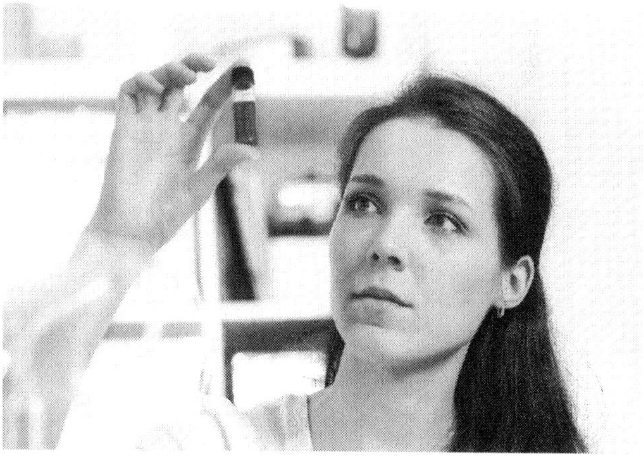

A1C Test (*Glycated Hemoglobin*) - This is the most common test used to determine most diabetes cases in the United States today. The test itself is a simple one. What it does is calculate the average blood sugar level in the body over the past two to three months. It will actually measure the amount of blood sugar that is currently attached to the rich, oxygen carrying protein in the red blood cells known as *haemoglobin*. With higher blood sugar saturation levels, the more of that protein will show up in the test.

These tests will be run more than once to guarantee accuracy. When two separate A1C tests come back with a level of 6.5 per cent or higher, the end result is diabetes. Anything between 6.4 per cent and 5.7 per cent is considered a high risk for developing diabetes in the future. However, anything lower than 5.7 per cent is considered normal blood sugar levels and thus, is healthy.

Unfortunately, there are times where the A1C test is not able to be run. These usually boil down to two groups: those that are pregnant and those that have an altered form of red blood cells known as haemoglobin variant. When either of those groups is present, one of three other tests will be used to determine diabetes.

Random Blood Sugar Test - Blood samples will be taken at a random time during the day. When levels of the random blood sugar test measure higher than 200 milligrams per decilitre of blood, it indicates diabetes. This, coupled with any symptoms of diabetes is usually a solid diagnosis. 199 milligrams to 140 milligrams are at high risk, and anything below 140 milligrams is again, healthy.

Fasting Blood Sugar Test - This is a simple test that allows a blood sample to be drawn after a basic overnight fasting period. When 126 milligrams of blood sugar shows up on two different tests, diabetes is diagnosed. Between 125 milligrams and 100 milligrams is the high risk range. And once again, below 100 milligrams is considered healthy.

Oral Glucose Tolerance Test - This test is rarely used anymore, as the other tests are far more reliable and easier to administer.

First, a patient will fast overnight and have a basic blood sugar level measured. After that, they will drink a sugary liquid. Once that is done, the blood sugar levels will be tested multiple times over two hours. When a reading of 200 milligrams or more comes up after those two hours, diabetes is diagnosed. 199 milligrams to 140 milligrams is once again at high risk. And of course, 140 milligrams and below means no diabetes.

Outside of direct testing for type 2 diabetes when the symptoms show up in any individual, the American Diabetes Association suggests that anyone that has reached the age of 45 be screened for type 2 diabetes every three years. This is even more important if you're overweight. Of course, anyone that is under 45 and still overweight should also be tested if other risk factors are present. These can include heart disease, a sedentary or lazy lifestyle, a personal history of gestational diabetes or a very high blood pressure. A family history of type 2 diabetes is also a great reason for getting yourself screened.

If diagnosed with diabetes, it is important to have your A1C levels checked at least twice a year. If possible, having the test run four times a year is even better. For most people, when they go in to have their A1C levels checked, they aim for a goal of 7 per cent or below. However, this number will vary from person to person, and should always be discussed with a doctor, preferably one that specializes in type 2 diabetes treatment.

While many people living with diabetes may wonder why they have to have these constant check-ups done when they're already checking their daily blood sugar at home, the answer is a simple one. The A1C testing is a much better indicator of just how well the treatment plan is progressing for individual care cases. When the A1C comes back elevated, it will naturally indicate that the treatment plan for the patient isn't working and needs to be changed.

So for anyone that has, or thinks they may have, diabetes, it is important to understand the tests involved so that they may better understand the disease itself. Please don't hesitate if you suspect that you're at risk.

Points to take away:

1) Whatever test your doctor recommends, just do it. It is vitally important to prevent future health problems.

Creating Your Custom Diabetes Diet Plan

Does having type 2 diabetes mean you will never enjoy food again?

No, of course not! This is the most common question I hear from newly diagnosed diabetics. You can still enjoy the yummiest foods and not feel deprived. You just have to know how to do it and perhaps make some adjustments in your perception of what is yummy!

I am not going to lay out a diet here complete with menus, because this will not benefit you. You're an individual and your diet must reflect your likes and dislikes as well as be based on your unique reaction to the foods you eat. If you're testing your glucose levels regularly, you're going to learn which foods cause a blood glucose spike and which foods you can eat more safely. What I *can* do is get you started by listing food types that are typically good for diabetes and those best avoided.

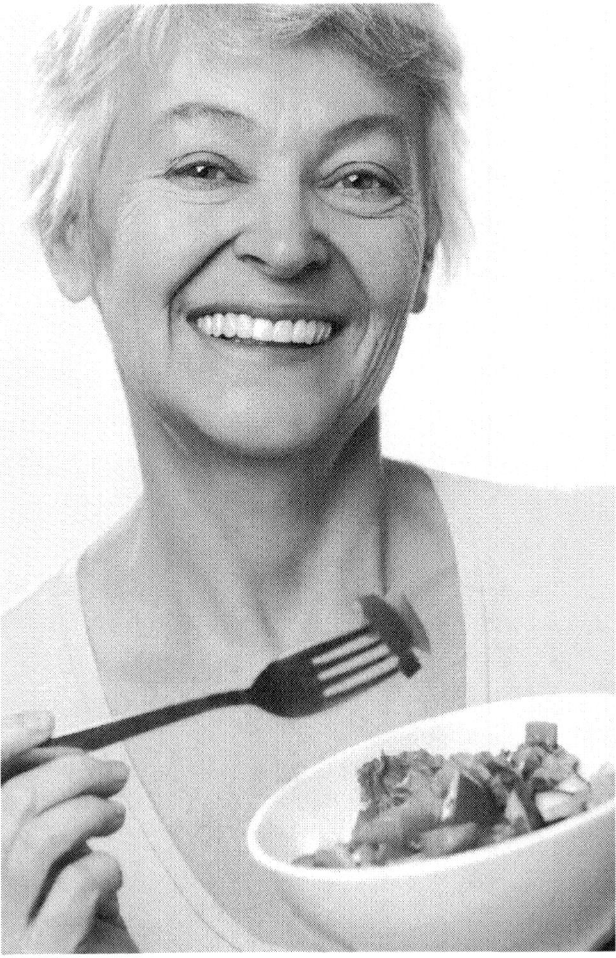

The foods you choose affect how your body functions

We know that too much glucose can trigger a multitude of health problems. The problem with most type 2 diabetics is not that they lack insulin; it's that their cells have become insulin resistant. This can mean that there may be too much insulin circulating in the blood stream.

Eating for type 2 diabetes is not just about trying to get serum glucose levels down. It's a question of balance. If your pancreas is happily producing insulin and the cells have become resistant to it, where is it going? It's going around in the blood stream and potentially causing havoc.

Too much insulin can cause *hypoglycaemia,* which means the level of glucose in the blood is too low. It can also cause other health problems such as auto immune diseases, vascular disease and cancer.

It's all about balance, you are constantly monitoring and balancing glucose and insulin levels. Yes it's very tedious! This is why you want to get rid of this disease as soon as possible. Meanwhile food can be your friend instead of your enemy.

The low carbohydrate diet

Current thinking is that everybody would be healthier on a low carbohydrate diet, not just those who suffer from, or who are at risk of, diabetes. The logic behind this is that humans did not start to cultivate grains until a long way into their evolutionary process. Hence the digestive system has not evolved sufficiently to properly digest grains, such as wheat, oats etc. Diabetics of course are forced to eat a controlled carbohydrate diet.

All carbohydrates are converted into glucose. However not all carbohydrates are equal. There are simple and complex carbohydrates. Loosely translated, simple carbohydrates are high GI - meaning they are converted into glucose very rapidly, whereas complex carbohydrates are low GI which take longer to convert to glucose. GI stands for the *glycaemic index* which is simply a measure of how fast different foods are converted into glucose.

What does this mean for the diabetic? When simple carbohydrates such as sugar or white rice are digested, glucose is formed very quickly, which triggers a large insulin release from the pancreas. The insulin then helps the cells to absorb this glucose for later release as energy. In type 2 diabetics, however, the cells are resistant to insulin and the glucose is not properly absorbed.

We already know all about what happens when there is constantly too much glucose in the bloodstream, so what happens when we eat complex carbohydrates, such as brown rice or a serve of broccoli? Glucose is released much more gradually with complex carbohydrates, allowing for less stress on the pancreas to produce a large amount of insulin.

So can diabetics eat carbohydrates and still keep their glucose levels down?

The short answer is, "Yes". The long answer is, "You need to manage it correctly".

If you have type 2 diabetes and want to manage it, you can still eat carbohydrates in moderation. If you want to lose weight in order to cure diabetes, it's best to give away the simple carbohydrates such as sugar (of all types) white bread and any baked goods made with white flour, white rice and highly processed foods.

Diabetes is reversible, but you can't go on eating the same way as you have been used to doing.

You can still eat whole grains such as wholemeal bread. However watch your portion sizes. You need fewer calories coming in than going out. This may seem awfully frustrating at first; however it's not too difficult. Here's how:

Eat regular meals at the same time each day

Try to regulate your meals at the same times during the day. Also try to keep meals around the same size. Don't have one huge meal for lunch and then have a few scraps for dinner. This will cause blood glucose swings. Some diabetics find eating five or six meals evenly spaced throughout the day helpful in maintaining glucose levels. Of course this is harder to do if you work full time.

Eat carbohydrates last

The easiest way to incorporate carbohydrates into a meal safely is to eat them last. Eat the protein (meat, fish eggs or chicken) first. What this will do is help prevent the rapid rise in blood sugar. It will also (in theory) probably mean you will eat less carbohydrate as you will feel fuller.

Like carbohydrate, protein is sometimes converted into glucose by a process called *gluconeogenesis*. The speed of this process is largely dependent on the amount of insulin secreted by the pancreas. But there is where the similarity ends.

Recent studies show that while an estimated 50% to 60% of protein could be converted to glucose, it does not enter the bloodstream and consequently does not raise the rate of glucose discharged by the liver. Protein is digested in the stomach and small intestine, whereas carbohydrates begin to be digested in the mouth.

The body will take its glucose from carbohydrates and will only take glucose from protein if the diet is carbohydrate free. This glucose would then be stored in the liver or muscles as glycogen. But experts agree that it is not likely to affect blood glucose levels.

Eat more fiber

People who are at risk of developing diabetes are advised to increase their fiber intake by taking fiber supplements such as *psyllium, guar gum, oat bran* or *glucomannan*. They should also consume more vegetables, fruits, whole wheat products and whole grain products. Eating fiber has a double benefit; because fiber is not actually digested, it can't add to the calorie (kilojoule) count. So you get to feel full without consuming extra calories.

However if you are used to a diet low in fiber, start adding it gradually over a couple of weeks. Otherwise you will be spending a lot of time in the bathroom!

Avoid highly processed foods

Highly processed foods are foods that have been altered significantly from their natural state. They include store bought cakes, cookies, instant meals, white flour, polenta, canned foods – the list goes on. Most foods that come in a package or a cardboard box will be processed to some degree. These foods are easily recognizable as they have a large list of ingredients on the package. Look at this and you're sure to find our old friend sugar in some form.

Sugar is added to savory as well as sweet foods to enhance flavor. This is an old trick. Increase the salt and sugar content and you can trick the taste buds. Avoid these types of foods.

Sugar can be disguised as corn syrup, cane juice, dextrose, maple syrup, malt syrup and sucrose. This is by no means a full list. See here for a complete list of sugar disguises.

http://www.hsph.harvard.edu/nutritionsource/added-sugar-on-food-labels/

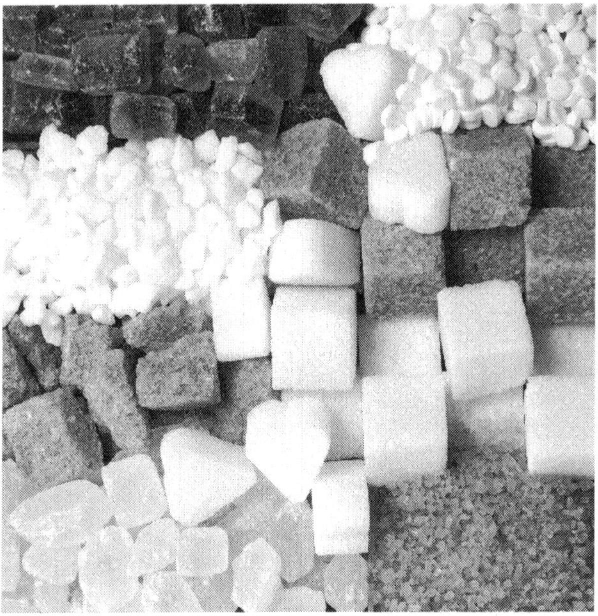

Some tips to help with your diabetes diet

Drink a glass of water before each meal. No it won't "dilute" your digestive juices, that is simply a myth. Squeeze some fresh lemon juice into the water and you've got yourself a great weight loss weapon that will lower the impact of carbohydrates. You'll get used to the taste and find it very refreshing. Although lemon juice is mildly acidic, it has an alkalizing effect in the body.

Sprinkle some vinegar on potatoes to lower the GI. If you love roast lamb, sprinkle mint sauce on your potato, it's made from vinegar.

Orange juice is very high in sugar and has barely any fiber. Eat your fruit whole instead.

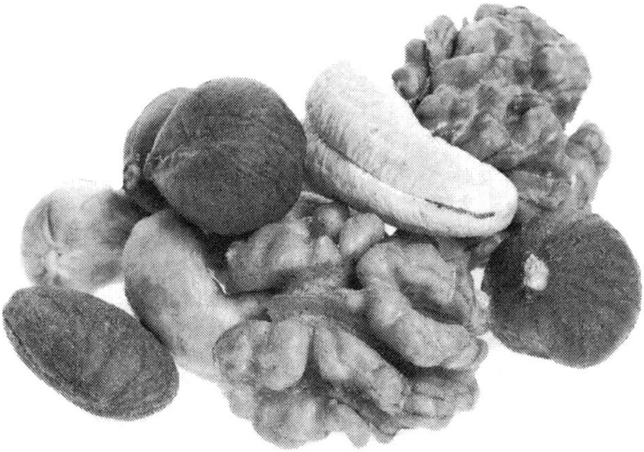

Snack on nuts if you're feeling hungry between meals. They contain vitamins and healthy fats, but make sure they are fresh. Keep them in the fridge to prevent them from going rancid. Nuts have properties which help the body use insulin and thus help insulin resistance.

Avocados are also great for glucose/insulin balance. Avocados are known to raise insulin sensitivity which helps cells better process blood glucose. They also contain healthy fats and will reduce your LDL (bad) cholesterol levels.

Don't be afraid of these natural fats, *they won't hurt you*. The fats you want to avoid are trans-fats found in margarine and many processed foods. Vegetable oils contain omega 6 which can upset the balance between omega 3 to omega 6 in the body. They also become toxic when heated to a high temperature.

The problem with vegetable oils is that they **sound** healthy. After all if something is made from vegetables it *should* be healthy. In fact just the opposite is true. Here are the real facts on these oils:

When referring to vegetable oils I'm talking about polyunsaturated oils, such as canola oil, safflower oil and sunflower oil. These artificially extracted oils can reduce

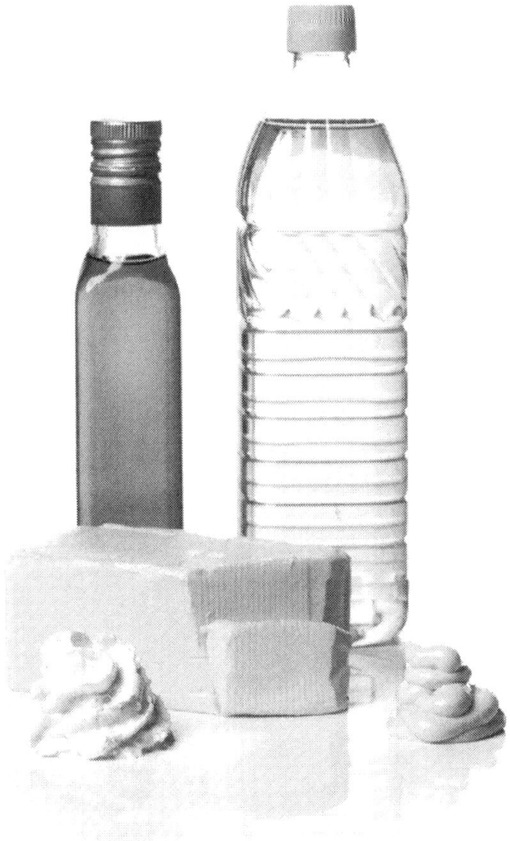

the cell's ability to absorb glucose thus making the cell more insulin resistant.

Polyunsaturated oils are chemically unstable and can also cause oxidation and the release of free radicals in the body. This can lead to further cell damage.

Olive oil is a *mono-saturated* oil which is good for the body. Olive oil can be safely used in salad dressings and some cooked dishes. It can destabilize at high temperatures so shouldn't be used for frying. Make sure that when you buy olive oil, you are getting the real thing and not a brand that has been diluted with an inferior polyunsaturated oil. This is happening a lot these days, so check the label carefully.

Coconut oil is fast being recognized as an unlikely health food due to its ability to remain stable at high temperatures which makes it highly suitable for frying and high temperature cooking.

Coconut oil also can help insulin production and can stabilize blood glucose levels, due to an ingredient called *Capric acid*.

There are many health benefits to this natural oil, especially if you're trying to lose weight. If you're interested you can find more information in The Coconut Oil Handbook - http://www.amazon.com/Coconut-Oil-miraculous-Beginners-ebook/dp/B00EP6M3VE/.

Butter has had a bad reputation due to the fact that it's a saturated fat. We have been taught that saturated fats are dangerous and can cause clogged arteries and heart problems. In fact this is completely false. Butter is a real food made without chemicals and the body recognizes it as such. Of course this is not a recommendation to slather a thick layer of butter on your food! Butter is still a fat and therefore high in calories.

However it is much better for your health than margarine when eaten in moderation. You only have to look back a couple of generations to see the truth about saturated fats. Our grandparents used butter and full cream milk, seemingly without any serious health issues. They even (shock horror!) used to cook in lard. Yet they were hardly affected by the diseases that plague us today.

Saturated fats also have certain health benefits. This type of fat facilitates calcium absorption for strong bones, protects the liver from toxins, helps brain and nerve function and can even improve metabolic function. The important thing to remember is moderation, especially when trying to lose weight.

Buckwheat is a grain which has been shown to lower glucose levels in various studies. Buckwheat contains an ingredient called *chiro-inositol* which is thought to stimulate the cells into being more insulin sensitive. Chiro-inositol is not found in any significant quantity in any other food.

Buckwheat is eaten extensively in some European countries. It can replace other grains in your diabetes meal plans and is definitely worth looking in to.

Beans - Although beans are a carbohydrate food, they contain many benefits for diabetics. This includes all types of beans, such as soy beans, navy beans and pinto beans. Even baked beans fit into this category, but watch out for high amounts of sugar and salt in the sauce. Beans contain a lot of soluble fiber, including pectin which binds to carbohydrates, slowing their digestion and preventing blood sugar swings.

Beans are high in protein and low in fat and can be made into a variety of meals, such as minestrone soup, dips, salads and Mexican cuisine. If using baked beans in cooking, rinse off the sauce before using.

Food Journal

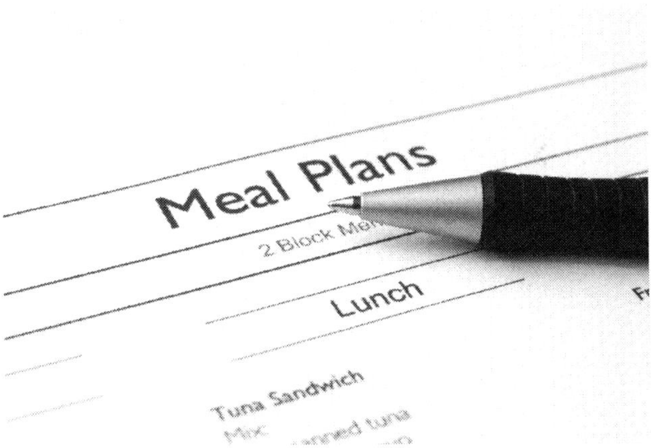

Keeping a food diary or journal is a great idea to keep a track of what you eat every day. Although this sounds pretty tedious, it can be a big help in pinpointing which foods affect your blood glucose levels more than others.

This can also be used as a reference to plan meals in advance. If you're also trying to lose weight and wondering why the pounds are not dropping off, a quick look at your food journal will probably give you a few clues.

Remember that your taste buds will change with time. If you can keep off the sweet foods for 28 days – the time it takes to change a habit – your desire for them WILL fade away. Along with the fat you've hated for so long.

A nutritionist can help

Of course if you don't feel confident setting up your own diet plan, a nutritionist can help. Nutritionists can recommend a customized starter plan for you, based on your own food preferences. You can always change it around at a later time, as long as you stick to the basic food groups. A nutritionist is skilled in food management and can be invaluable when it comes to weight loss.

Mindset

If you can get your mind to work for, instead of against you, you can make positive changes much more easily. You won't feel deprived or depressed, which is why we're going to look at mindset in the next chapter.

Points to take away:

1) Change the way you look at food. It's there to nourish your body, not to reward yourself with. You can still enjoy food without being addicted to it.

2) You don't have to totally give up carbohydrates, just manage them better.

3) Space your meals out evenly through the day.

4) Avoid dangerous fats such as trans-fats and poly-unsaturated vegetable oils. Use butter, olive oil and coconut oil in moderation instead.

5) Get sugar out of your diet. It's totally do-able and you'll feel a lot better. Remember 28 days - starting today!

How to Have a Positive Mindset

It's all in the mind! How to get your mind working for you.

You are about to change some bad habits for better ones. Breaking bad habits isn't easy. It takes a lot of repetition for an action to become a habit. Why do we repeat certain behaviors? It's because they serve some useful function in our lives.

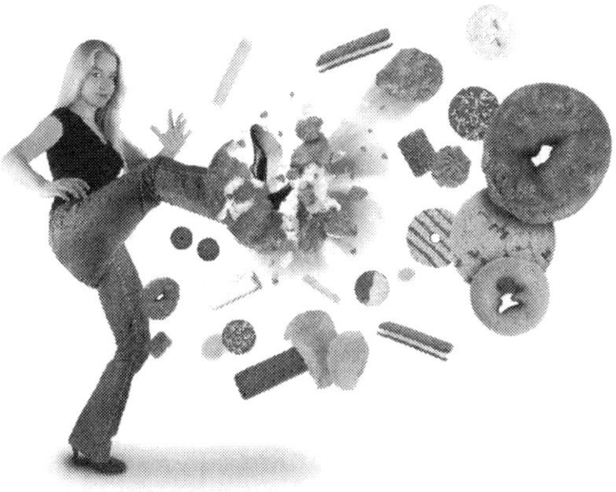

Let's look at food first. In theory we eat because we are hungry. Our body sends us hunger signals on a regular basis. This is programmed into our brain and is controlled by certain hormones. If we did not receive these hunger signals and forgot to eat, we would have no energy, our bodies would not repair themselves and we would eventually die.

The trouble is, *hunger is not the only reason we eat*. We may eat because we are bored, upset, happy, depressed or simply because we know there is a bar of our favorite chocolate sitting in the cupboard!

We use food as a drug to soothe our troubled minds. Some people use alcohol, some people use prescription drugs or tobacco. Other people have a healthier way of dealing with troublesome emotions, they exercise. However healthy this choice may seem, exercising can also be overdone.

Adding to this problem is the fact that sugar is addictive, in fact some health experts claim it can be as addictive as tobacco for some individuals.

While that may be true, it doesn't take as long to get rid of a sugar addiction as it does a smoking habit (I know because I had one).

So eating sweet pleasant tasting foods is actually helping us deal with unpleasant emotions and that's why it has become a habit. Can you find another outlet for these emotions? Here are a few suggestions to try:

1) Write out what's bothering you on a piece of paper (typing into a document doesn't work as well). Read it through then tear it up and throw it away. This gets the problem out of your mind and onto paper. The act of tearing it up and throwing it away send a message to your subconscious mind to let that problem go.

2) Talk to a friend about your problem. This also "gets it out there". Other people may be able to offer suggestions you may never have thought of by yourself.

3) Try EFT. This stands for Emotional Freedom Technique. This is a simple self-help technique you can use to banish

negative thoughts, heal old emotional wounds from childhood, eliminate stress and cure cravings. You simply tap on certain acupressure points on the body to get relief.

EFT is fast growing in popularity around the world. Of course it is an alternative therapy, so don't ask your doctor about it, you'll probably get a blank stare! Below is a link to some resources you can check out if you're interested.

EFT is free, you can use it whenever you want and it flat out **works**.

http://www.eftuniverse.com/tutorial/learn-eft

Here is a quick little EFT routine to deal with sudden cravings. This is only a temporary fix, but it can get you past the bakery safely!

Tap lightly with two fingers using either hand. Tap 5-6 times on each point:

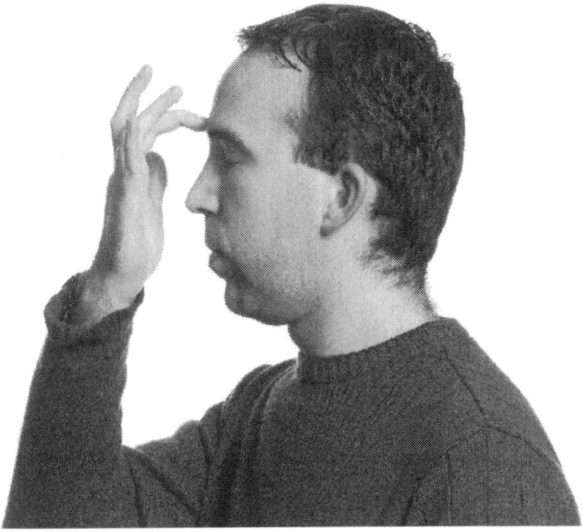

- On the bottom of the eye socket, just under the eye
- Around 4 inches below your underarm
- On your collarbone (just to the side of and underneath the bone itself)

You can just repeat the tapping until the craving is gone. There are no side effects to this technique, although you might feel a slight energy shift. This is normal and good.

Some of our food habits started in early childhood. Were you told you had to finish everything on your plate before you could leave the table? You may still be doing this even though you're no longer hungry. You can choose to be aware of these old habits and let them go.

Do you eat while watching TV? You may not be conscious of becoming full and this can bypass your natural appetite control. Always eat with awareness.

How large is your plate? Try using the same amount of food on a smaller plate. This is telling your subconscious mind there is a lot of food on your plate and you'll feel full sooner. This is a mind trick, but it works well.

Don't beat yourself up if you occasionally make the wrong food choices. Just accept that you're human and move on. No-one is perfect; you can only do your best.

Learn to love exercise

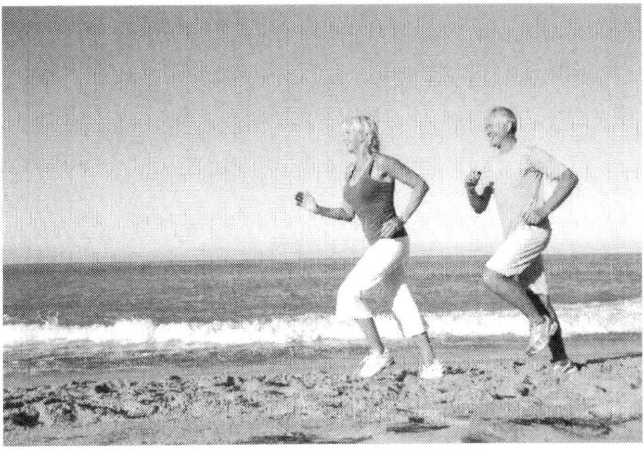

Why don't we exercise when we know we should? In this case it's because doing nothing is easier than getting up and moving. If running or walking is your exercise of choice, it may be that the weather's awful and you can't get out, you may be too busy to exercise or you may simply forget.

Eventually you get tired of feeling guilty and rationalize that exercise doesn't really burn that many calories anyway! Why not just cut down on our afternoon snack and have one cookie instead of two?

Our minds are very clever at finding reasons not to do something that we don't feel like doing. If you're aware of this you're half way to fixing it. If you really want to cure type 2 diabetes, you have to adopt better eating and exercise habits and it won't be easy at first. However, keep a picture firmly in your mind of a slim, healthier you and your mind will then steer you towards that reality.

Use the power of your mind to work for you instead of against you. The mind should be your servant, not your master. Show it who's in charge!

We all have problems. What may seem like an insurmountable problem today, you might not even remember a year from now. Re-frame your problems as challenges and look at them as opportunities to find a better way to do things.

Points to take away

1) Try not to focus on what you are giving up, but what you are gaining.

2) We can use food as a drug when we're upset or bored. Be aware of this and find other outlets for your negative emotions. EFT is great for this.

3) Don't beat yourself up if you make a mistake. Just forgive yourself and move on.

4) You are a special person and you deserve to be healthy!

I Hate Exercise Can I Make it Easier?

Exercise - It makes you feel good!

This is probably going to be a short chapter. Why? Because the good news is ANY kind of exercise you do will benefit you on so many levels. Not only will you burn fat, but you'll improve your body's ability to absorb glucose into the muscles. There are many other benefits to regular exercise, such as lowering blood pressure, improving mood and strengthening your bones and muscles.

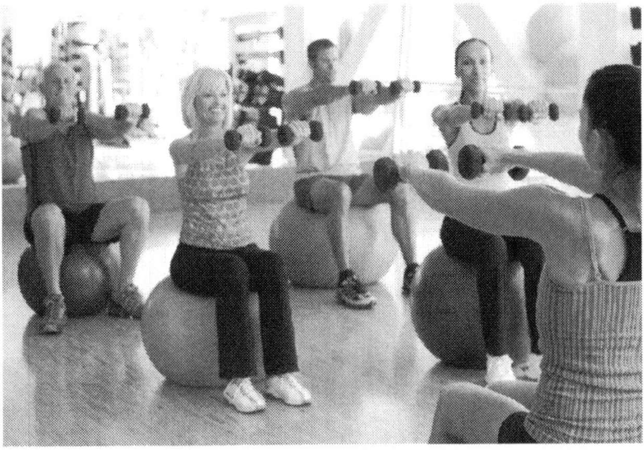

The beauty of exercise is the effects can last up to 24 hours after you have finished. Blood glucose levels will stay lower for longer.

There is a specific type of exercise which will help you lose weight a lot faster too, but we'll get to that a bit later...

The worst thing you can do if you've not exercised in a long while is to suddenly jump into a vigorous exercise routine. You'll end up stiff and sore and probably hate the thought of exercising for ever more.

Just start gently. The best thing is to try and do a little exercise every day. To start with you can fit this into your everyday routine by walking to the next bus stop, walking to the shops, climbing the stairs instead of taking the lift or taking a walk in your lunch break. Make a list of the ways you can include more movement into your day.

As you become a bit fitter, you could make yourself a diabetes exercise plan to suit your lifestyle. To keep yourself motivated, make out a list of goals to aim for, such as losing a certain amount of weight by Christmas or fitting into that favorite pair of jeans again.

Keep your goals realistic and remember to reward yourself when you achieve your target. It could be a nice trip away or some nice clothes. No a box of chocolates is not an option!

Choosing an exercise that you enjoy will ensure you can stick to your exercise goals. Nothing is worse than trying to force yourself to do something you don't enjoy. Try swimming laps, walking, jogging or any exercise that can raise your heart rate for at least 10 minutes or more.

Aim for 30 minutes of aerobic exercise three or four times a week. This could be brisk walking, swimming, cycling or jogging. This will increase your heart rate and get those muscles using up that glucose. If you're very unfit, start with 10 minutes and build up to 30.

On the days that you're not doing aerobic exercise, see if you can fit in some Yoga or Pilates. If you don't want to go to a class, or there's nothing in your area, there are some great exercise DVDs you can buy. There's no need for expensive gym memberships or fancy machines; getting fit can be done without spending any money on equipment. The one exception to this is a good pair of walking shoes.

If you like the idea of using weights to increase muscle mass, (both girls and guys can do this) use soup cans, or for guys, fill empty plastic containers with sand or water and get pumping! Girls you will not end up with huge muscles, just nicely toned arms. Increasing muscle mass will really help the glucose absorption too.

One thing to remember is to test your glucose levels before and after exercising as exercise can both increase or decrease your levels in the short term. Don't exercise if your glucose levels are over 250-300 mg/dL (or 16.7 mmol/L). This means you have a high level of ketones and exercising at these levels can cause a serious side effect called *ketoacidosis*. (MayoClinic.com)

Exercise for fat loss.

This may not appeal to everyone, but it can reduce weight faster than normal aerobic exercise. You can do this on a stationary bike, a real bike or simply walking along the road. The aim is to fit intense activity in between slow bouts of activity.

For example cycle slowly for 2 minutes, then as fast as you can for 30 seconds, then slow down for 90 seconds before speeding up again for 30 seconds. After around 10 minutes of this you will have burned off around the same number of calories as 90 minutes of normal aerobic exercise.

If this is too strenuous, simply walk slowly and then walk fast or do a slow jog for 10 seconds. You can adapt this to fit in with your fitness level.

WARNING – This is not for those who have never exercised or who are very unfit. Also always check with your doctor before starting any type of exercise other than just walking.

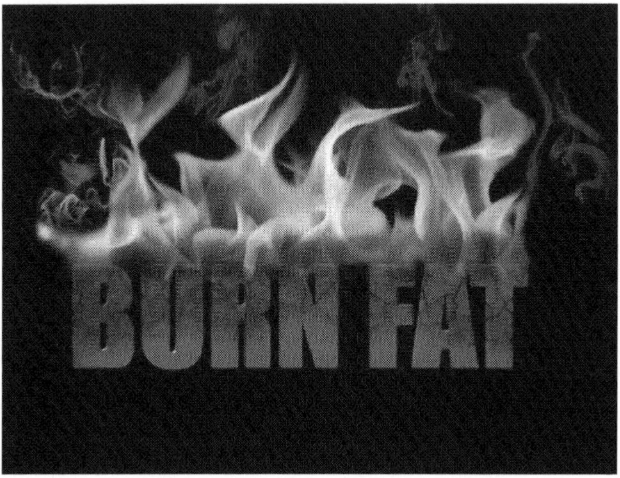

It takes a while to start really enjoying exercise, but you will find, the longer you persevere, the more you will like it, so keep going!

Points to take away:

1) Start any exercise routine slowly, don't push yourself too hard.

2) Even though you may not believe it, you will get to enjoy exercise as it becomes a habit.

3) Don't forget to test those glucose levels.

Combating Type 2 Diabetes with Natural Supplements

Natural Remedies for Diabetes

Living with type 2 diabetes is no fun for anyone. But there are ways to make it a lot easier.

Naturally, eating the right food and taking the proper medication, (when necessary) is paramount, but is there anything else we can do to make life easier?

Indeed there is! There are herbs and natural supplements available that can help diabetics tremendously. Not all of them will work for you, but most diabetics can benefit from at least one of these remedies and sometimes the benefits are surprising.

So here is a natural supplement list that can help the symptoms of type 2 diabetes and actually make your life a lot easier as you are heading towards a cure. While there are no substitutes for proper diet and exercise, these natural supplements make a great addition to the diet of any type 2 diabetic.

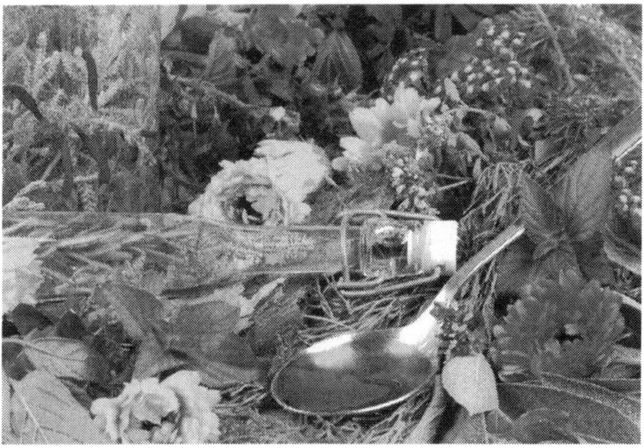

Gymnema Sylvestre

Out of the Indian forests comes possibly the best supplement for diabetes and pre-diabetes, *Gymnema Sylvestre.* This Ayurvedic remedy can even improve the symptoms of type 1 diabetes. It has three specific benefits:

1) Controls sugar cravings.
2) Helps cells better absorb glucose, and
3) Increases pancreatic release of insulin

The active ingredient is *gymnemic acid* (a *saponin*) which suppresses our ability to taste sweet foods. The beneficial effects were first discovered in the 1920s.

There are documented cases of people who have been able to give up their type 2 diabetes medications after taking Gymnema for a few weeks. (Journal of Ethnopharmacology – October 1990) The recommended daily dose of Gymnema is 400 mg per day. It is possible to take more, but consult with your health practitioner first.

Coffee Berry

Coffee berry actually stimulates the beta cells in the pancreas. Not only does the coffee berry help give a nice boost to beta cell activity and insulin production, but it will also help reduce free radicals in the body and actually help support optimal blood glucose levels throughout the body, making it a win-win situation for any diabetic. But it is important to note that just because coffee beans come from coffee berries, a cup of joe in the morning isn't going to give you these benefits! Instead, stick with a coffee berry supplement that will provide all of the healthy nutrients that are destroyed when the bean is dry roasted after being removed from the fruit.

Chlorogenic and Caffeic Acid

These two acids, when taken in supplement form, help diabetics in one very distinct way - glucose management. *Chlorogenic* acid supplements actually help restrict the formation of glucose in the bloodstream by basically blocking the production of the enzyme that allows it. It also hinders the transport of glucose by stopping it from being absorbed into the blood itself.

Caffeic acid on the other hand, actually increases the glucose uptake into the cells themselves. This helps remove excess blood sugar from the bloodstream, helping reduce the blood glucose levels of any diabetic. When combined, the effect that these two acid supplements have on the blood sugar level is a marvellous one indeed.

Cinnamon

Who doesn't love a little cinnamon in their morning cereal? Used throughout the world to treat many different ailments, it should be no surprise that cinnamon can also help type 2 diabetics looking for natural ways to balance their blood glucose. Cinnamon can be added to many other foods for flavor, and has the added benefit of lowering blood glucose. It contains natural compounds that can mimic insulin, which give it many benefits for diabetics.

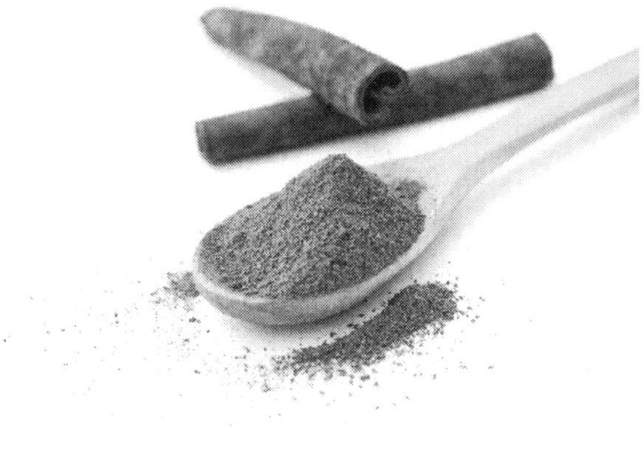

Cinnamon actually has the ability to help increase the body's ability to metabolize glucose. This in turn will help reduce the insulin resistance that is the core cause of type 2 diabetes. Due to the other natural benefits of cinnamon, the reduction in lipid levels combined with the benefits for type 2 diabetes actually increases heart health and helps reduce the risk of cardiovascular disease. As cardiovascular disease is common in diabetic people, this is yet another win-win situation that can be found simply by embracing the power of cinnamon in the diet.

Store bought cinnamon can contain little of the active ingredient though. There are many supplements out there with the same *polyphenols* found in cinnamon that will do a better job. Many health food stores will also sell cinnamon supplements, which are basically the extracted polyphenols and other healthy aspects of cinnamon all crammed into a tiny pill to help embrace all the benefits of cinnamon without actually altering your diet.

Bitter melon

Also known as *Mamordica Charantia,* bitter melon is a vegetable containing *saponins, alkaloids* and *peptides* that combine to significantly enhance the action of beta cells in the pancreas, thus improving insulin production. Bitter melon originates from the Philippines where it is used as a natural supplement and is also popular in Chinese medicine.

As the name suggests this vegetable is bitter! However it is also available in capsule form.

Gogi Berries

Sufferers of type 2 diabetes may already know that blurred vision is a major curse caused by the increased blood sugar levels actually leeching the fluids out of the lenses in the eyes. Since visual impairment is something that nobody needs, finding a natural supplement that can be taken to help combat that is a huge bonus.

And that is exactly what *gogi berries* and their extract can offer. By taking gogi berry extract, you can lower the oxidative stress that the eyes are subjected to during type 2 diabetes, essentially lowering the strain on the eye and helping to correct vision impairment problems caused by high blood glucose levels.

Vitamin D

Vitamin D occurs naturally in the body from the action of sunlight on skin. Besides having numerous health benefits, a lack of vitamin D has been associated with higher prevalence of type 2 diabetes. Although not clinically proven, small studies have consistently found those with lower levels of this vitamin appear have a greater incidence of type 2 diabetes. Those most at risk of being deficient in vitamin D are people with dark skins and those who work indoors and are therefore not exposed to the sun.

Supplements of vitamin D are readily available, but it's best to check levels first with your next blood test. Vitamin D is a fat soluble vitamin and as such, can be toxic in large doses. Naturally formed vitamin D from exposure to sunlight is preferable if you can get outdoors daily.

Minerals

Minerals are inorganic substances usually found in small amounts naturally in the body. Although they are only needed in small amounts, deficiencies can severely affect our health. Those that help with diabetes are:

Magnesium – helps with insulin production in diabetics. Many people, particularly diabetics, are low in this mineral. Magnesium is also beneficial for heart health. Magnesium is poorly absorbed by the body. There trans-dermal sprays which can now be purchased that are better absorbed.

Potassium – Potassium levels are usually low in those with type 2 diabetes; possibly due to high protein intake. Good source of potassium are bananas and citrus fruits.

Chromium Picolinate - This is a trace mineral that can help with those pesky sugar cravings. Chromium can also help metabolize carbohydrates and help with glucose absorption.

Be aware that overdoses of these minerals can be dangerous – especially potassium. Always check the dosage on the label.

Myo-inositol - Sometimes known as vitamin B8, this substance can be useful for *diabetic neuropathy*. Low levels of Myo-inositol have been found in those with neuropathy. It can be found in whole grains and legumes and also available as supplements.

Vitamin B12 is another vitamin that can help with diabetic neuropathy. This is particularly important for vegetarians who are commonly low in this vitamin. Deficiency in B12 can cause nervous system damage.

It could be a good idea for diabetics to take a good Vitamin B complex tablet daily, preferably one that is food based, if they suffer with diabetic neuropathy.

Anti-oxidants

Anti-oxidants are necessary in everyone's diet as they combat free radicals caused by oxidative stress. Free radicals cause tissue damage in the body because they carry an extra negatively charged electron which tries to attach to cells, causing havoc in the process.

Complications from diabetes are further enhanced by these free radicals. Therefore *anything* that can be done to minimize damage to the body's tissues is paramount.

There are many anti-oxidants available, both in the diet and as supplements. Brightly colored fruits and vegetables are typically high in anti-oxidants. Choose berries (especially blueberries), citrus fruits, tomatoes, red beans and red bell peppers. Anti-oxidant supplements are available, but don't seem as effective as those obtained fresh from food.

As you can see, there are many natural supplements that are available to help to cope with living with diabetes. Together with a sensible diet and healthy lifestyle, using the above supplements can help fight diabetes. While changing your entire world to revolve around a proper diet and exercise can be difficult for anyone, using quality supplements can help get you through the day.

Points to take away:

1) There are supplements such as herbs and vitamins that have a beneficial effect on type 2 diabetes.

2) Anti-oxidants may be taken in supplemental form but are better sourced from fresh fruit and vegetables and brightly colored foods.

Appendix 1 - Artificial and Natural Sweeteners

To use or not to use? That is the question.

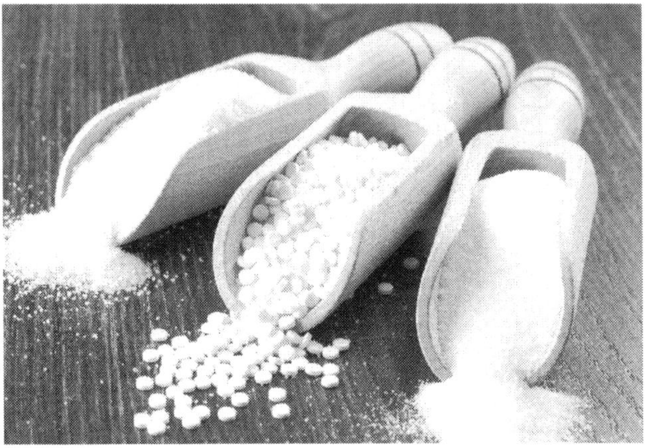

If sugar is off the menu, it would probably make sense to use artificial sweeteners instead, wouldn't it?

Here's the thing. Most artificial sweeteners have zero calories and they don't cause a spike in insulin. That's the good news.

Here's the bad news. They are all chemicals and they could have health implications in the long term. The other piece of bad news, which is backed up by many scientific studies, is that people who use artificial sweeteners gain more weight than those who use sugar.

This seems to make no sense at all and until recently, no-one was sure why this was the case. It's because the body's sense of taste gets confused when consuming a chemically sweetened food.

The digestive system prepares for a high calorie load and when this doesn't happen it affects the natural appetite control center of the brain. It also affects the metabolic reaction to food, meaning you expend fewer calories.

More deadly than this, however, is the destructive effect of some of these chemical sweeteners on your body. There are several different types of sweeteners on the market today and some are worse than others when it comes to your health. Particularly bad are those made with a chemical called *Aspartame.*

NutraSweet

NutraSweet is made from *aspartame* and should be avoided at all costs. Aspartame is the most controversial of all the artificial sweeteners on the market. Its side effects can fill a whole book.

Having said that, there is indeed such a book written about the dreadful side effects of this chemical. Called "*Aspartame Disease: An Ignored Epidemic*" by Dr H J Roberts M.D. It outlines the deadly effects of consuming aspartame. The deadly side effects are numerous and if I were to list them all here, this book would never be finished!

Here are a few of the documented effects of aspartame – muscle cramps, pain, convulsions, abdominal pain, slurred speech, memory loss, fatigue, increased hunger and cancer. Would you like a teaspoon of NutraSweet in your coffee? I think not!

Equal and Canderel®

More brand names based on aspartame. Thus the above warnings and side effects apply.

Splenda

Notice how splendid some of these name are? The manufacturers have gone to some trouble to make them sound wholesome and healthy! Splenda, however fails to live up to its illustrious title. Splenda's main ingredient is *Sucralose,* which claims to made from sugar. In fact it has a similar chemical structure and flavor, but that's where the similarity ends. Sucralose contains chlorine which is carcinogenic and can have numerous side effects including depression, mood swings, skin rashes and digestive problems.

Splenda also contains *dextrose* and *maltodextrin*. It does contain fewer calories than sugar, but does contain carbohydrates. With all that going for it, why would you bother?

Sweet'N Low

Sweet'N Low is based on *saccharin*. Saccharin has been around since the early 1900s, which gives it the advantage that it has stood the test of time.

Saccharin is an extremely sweet substance with a slightly bitter after taste. This is still a chemical substance, but probably not as dangerous as aspartame. It can cause allergies, headaches and stomach upsets. Saccharin is not digested and, as such, doesn't enter the bloodstream.

Hermesetas

Hermesetas is another brand name based mainly on saccharin.

Sweet One

Sweet One is based on the substance *Acesulfame K*. Acesulfame K is 200 times sweeter than sugar and has not undergone rigorous testing, so not too much is known about its effects. There are side effects that are coming to light though; Acesulfame K may cause nausea, headaches, mood swings, damage to the organs, such as the liver and kidneys, vision problems and possibly even cancer. Approach with caution!

Natural Sweeteners

Natural sweeteners come with many of the advantages of artificial sweeteners, but without many of the dangers. However some of these do contain calories and carbohydrates. Unfortunately there is no perfect answer to a sweet tooth!

Stevia

Most natural health gurus recommend this herbal sweetener. I have tried to like the taste of Stevia but have given up. It has an aftertaste that follows you around all day! Try it by all means; it is a much healthier option than the chemical sweeteners. Some people like it. Personally I would rather have no sweetener at all.

Xylitol

Xylitol is one of the better known "wood alcohols"; *Sorbitol* is another. These natural sweeteners are made from wood, corn or other fibrous plants. Xylitol tastes like sugar and can be used for sweetening drinks or for cooking.

Xylitol is not completely calorie free; it has just over half the calories of sugar. However it is low in carbohydrate content, having a GI of just 7. This makes it much more suitable for diabetics, as the sudden release of insulin is not triggered.

Xylitol has the added benefit of being an anti-bacterial substance. It inhibits tooth decay and may also inhibit other dangerous bacteria in the body.

Is there a downside to using Xylitol? It is quite expensive to buy compared with natural sugar. Also side effects can include bloating and diarrhea, due to the fact it is digested in the intestines. I use Xylitol to sweeten my tea and find that by trying different brands, those symptoms can be avoided; however some people can't tolerate it at all. People suffering from epilepsy should also avoid this product as it can contribute to seizures. It is also very toxic for dogs.

Coconut sugar

Coconut sugar is made from the sap of the coconut tree blossoms. The liquid is first collected into containers and then placed under heat until the water has all evaporated. This leaves a crystalline substance which is known as coconut sugar.

Coconut sugar does have some nutritious substances in it, for example potassium, zinc and calcium and it also contains traces of antioxidants. The most interesting ingredient however is a fiber called *Inulin*. This is thought to slow down the absorption of glucose and could well be why coconut sugar has a much lower GI than regular sugar. Regular sugar has a GI of around 60 were as coconut sugar is around 35.

Despite the fact that it contains traces of nutrients, coconut sugar at the end of the day, is still a sugar and has roughly the same number of calories. Although it has a lower GI, it should be limited in the diet.

Points to take away:

1) There is always a danger to your health from consuming artificial substances. Particularly avoid sweeteners containing aspartame.

2) Xylitol is probably an option for some as it has a low carbohydrate count. Stevia is also a healthy option, but has an unpleasant aftertaste.

3) The ideal answer is to train your taste buds to not crave sweet foods. This is possible to do, but not easy! Try doing it gradually.

4) If you **must** use an artificial sweetener, a saccharin based sweetener such as Sweet'N Low would probably be your safest option.

Conclusion

I hope that you have enjoyed this book and that it can help you win the battle against type 2 diabetes.

If you are on medication for diabetes, it is very important not to stop taking this without consulting your doctor or health provider.

Yes, diabetes can be reversed by eating well, losing weight and exercising, but do not stop your medication or glucose testing without being cleared by your doctor first. This is crucial!

I would like to hear your success story! If you feel this book has helped you, please let me know. That was why this book was written, in the hope that in some small way it could stem the tide of the ever growing diabetes epidemic.

I wish you a long, healthy and happy life!

26619813R00063

Printed in Great Britain
by Amazon